THE MENOPAUSE GUIDE

Empowering your journey through Hormonal changes with science and strength.

Berta J.stewart

Acknowledgements

Expressing "The Menopause Guide" has been a mind boggling excursion, and I'm profoundly thankful to the numerous people who have upheld and propelled me en route. Above all else, I need to thank the endless ladies who imparted their own accounts and encounters to menopause. Your fortitude, trustworthiness, and versatility have been a steady wellspring of motivation and have significantly molded the substance of this book. To my family, particularly my mate, your relentless help and understanding have been my stone. Much thanks to you for your understanding during the late evenings and long days of composing, and for continuously putting stock in my vision. I owe a colossal obligation of appreciation to my companions and partners in the ladies' wellbeing local area. Your mastery, input, and support have been priceless. on account of Anna j . Smith,whose experiences and direction have improved this book in endless ways. I'm likewise profoundly thankful to the scientists and medical services experts whose work on menopause has established the groundwork for this aide. Your commitments to the field are key, and I'm regarded to expand upon your insight. In conclusion, to each peruser holding this book: much obliged. Your obligation to understanding and embracing this phase of life is both rousing and lowering. I trust "The Menopause Guide" fills in as a significant asset and wellspring of help on your excursion. With appreciation. Berta j.stewart.

About the author

Berta J. Stewart is a devoted backer for ladies' wellbeing, dedicated to enabling ladies to explore life's changes with certainty and elegance. With a significant enthusiasm for aiding ladies comprehend and embrace the progressions that accompany menopause, Berta has turned into a confident voice in the field of ladies' wellbeing and health. Much thanks to you for getting some margin to peruse "The Menopause Guide." It is Berta's expectation that this book fills in as an important asset and wellspring of motivation for ladies all over. Keep in mind, menopause is an excursion — that you don't need to walk alone. Together, we can explore this progress with strength, elegance, and a restored feeling of direction.

Table of contents

Introduction

Whenever I first felt it, I was always in line at the supermarket. One second, I was flipping through a magazine, and the following, a rush of intensity flooded through my body, leaving me flushed and dazed. Maybe an undetectable switch had been flipped, and I was unable to stop it. I fanned myself with the magazine, humiliated and somewhat frightened. Was this what menopause felt like? I had heard stories from companions and read articles, however nothing had set me up for the truth. It was then that I understood how little I had some awareness of this huge period of life, and the amount I really wanted an aide — something exhaustive, functional, and compassionate. That is the reason I chose to state "The Menopause Guide." Menopause is a characteristic piece of life, yet it remains covered in secret and misinterpretations. For some ladies, the progress is loaded with tension and disarray. In any case, it doesn't need to be like this. This guide is here to change that story, to offer lucidity and solace, and to act as a confided in friend through each phase of menopause. Whether you're simply starting to see the signs or are very much into your postmenopausal years, this book is intended to enable you with information and backing. We'll begin by demystifying what menopause is and what it isn't. Disregard the fantasies and shocking tales; menopause isn't the finish of your lively life yet another part with its own one of a kind difficulties and potential open doors. In Section 1, "Grasping Menopause," we'll dive into the natural cycles behind this progress. You'll find out about the hormonal changes that trigger menopause, the various stages (perimenopause, menopause, and postmenopause), and what's in store at each stage. Information is power, and understanding what's going on in your body can assist you with exploring this excursion with certainty.

Early signs and side effects can be dumbfounding, yet admonished is forearmed. In Part 2, "Early Signs and Side effects," we'll investigate the normal pointers that menopause is drawing closer. From hot glimmers and night sweats to mind-set swings and unpredictable periods, we'll cover everything. You'll track down point by point clarifications for every side effect, alongside pragmatic ways to oversee them. It's tied in with assuming command over your experience, as opposed to allowing it to control you. Hormonal changes are at the core of menopause, influencing everything from your rest examples to your close to home prosperity. In Section 3, "Hormonal Changes," we'll separate these mind boggling processes into reasonable terms. You'll find what estrogen and progesterone vacillations mean for your body and psyche, and how you might adjust these changes. We'll examine both normal cures and clinical medicines, providing you with a full range of choices to consider. Overseeing menopause doesn't need to depend entirely on clinical intercessions. Section 4, "Overseeing Side effects Normally," is committed to all encompassing methodologies that can have a massive effect. We'll cover the significance of diet and sustenance, the advantages of normal activity, and the mending force of home grown cures. We'll likewise present pressure to the executives strategies like care and yoga, which can work on your general personal satisfaction.

Clinical therapies, including Chemical Substitution Treatment (HRT), have their place as well, and in Section 5, "Clinical Medicines," we'll give a reasonable perspective on these choices. You'll find out about the advantages and dangers of HRT, non-hormonal prescriptions, and elective treatments. This part means to outfit you with the data expected to settle on informed choices in conference with your medical services supplier. Your psychological and close to home prosperity are similarly basically as significant as your actual wellbeing. In Part 6, "Mental and Profound Prosperity," we'll address the mental effect of menopause. From adapting to nervousness and misery to keeping up with mental wellbeing, this section offers systems for remaining intellectually and genuinely adjusted. We'll likewise examine the significance of a solid encouraging group of people and looking for proficient assistance when required. Menopause can influence your personal connections as well. In Section 7, "Sexual Wellbeing," we'll discuss changes in moxie, vaginal wellbeing, and how to keep up with closeness with your accomplice. Fair correspondence and commonsense exhortation can assist you with exploring this delicate region with certainty and empathy. Long haul wellbeing contemplations become really squeezing post-menopause. Part 8, "Long haul Wellbeing," centers around issues like bone thickness and osteoporosis, cardiovascular wellbeing, weight of the board, and changes in skin and hair. Preventive measures and solid way of life decisions can essentially affect your prosperity in the years to come.

Menopause is an excursion that each lady sets out on, yet with the right data and backing, it very well may be an excursion of strengthening and self-revelation. This guide plans to be your confidant friend, offering astuteness, down to earth counsel, and consolation constantly. Together, we'll explore this progress with effortlessness, strength, and certainty. Welcome to "The Menopause Guide." How about we leave on this excursion together..

Chapter 1:

Understanding Menopause

Definition and Stages

Menopause is a characteristic natural cycle that denotes the finish of a lady's conception years. It is characterized as the discontinuance of feminine periods for 12 back to back months, commonly happening between the ages of 45 and 55. Notwithstanding, the experience of menopause is exceptionally individual and can shift generally from one lady to another. Menopause is comprehensively partitioned into three phases: Perimenopause: This is the momentary period paving the way to menopause. It can start quite a long while before menopause, as the ovaries slowly produce less estrogen. During this stage, ladies might begin to encounter sporadic feminine cycles and different side effects, for example, hot glimmers and emotional episodes. Menopause: This stage is formally reached when a lady has gone a year without a feminine period. The ovaries quit delivering eggs, and there is a huge drop in the creation of estrogen and progesterone. Postmenopause: This stage starts following menopause and go on until the end of a lady's life. Side effects like hot glimmers might endure, however they by and large abatement in power and recurrence over the long run. The concentration during this stage is in many cases on overseeing long haul wellbeing chances related with the reduction in estrogen levels, like osteoporosis and coronary illness. The Menopausal Change The menopausal change, otherwise called perimenopause, can be a difficult time for some ladies. Portrayed by critical hormonal changes can cause a great many physical and close to home side effects. Understanding these progressions can assist you with overseeing them all the more actually.

During perimenopause, the degrees of estrogen and progesterone created by the ovaries vary capriciously. This can prompt changes in feminine cycle designs, remembering varieties for cycle length, missed periods, and changes in feminine stream. A few ladies may likewise encounter side effects, for example, hot blazes, night sweats, rest unsettling influences, and emotional episodes. These hormonal changes are a typical piece of maturing and mean the body's progress away from conceptive capability. While the side effects can be awkward, they are commonly brief and can be dealt with way of life changes and clinical medicines. Normal Side effects Menopause is in many cases joined by different side effects, some of which can altogether affect day to day existence. Here are probably the most widely recognized side effects: Hot Blazes: Unexpected sensations of serious intensity, frequently joined by perspiring and a quick heartbeat. Hot glimmers can endure from a couple of moments to a few minutes and can happen on various occasions a d myay. Night Sweats: Extreme hot blazes that happen during rest and can prompt critical inconvenience and rest aggravations. Sporadic Periods: Changes in feminine cycle length, stream, and recurrence are normal during perimenopause. Rest Aggravations: Trouble nodding off or staying unconscious, frequently because of night sweats or tension. Mind-set Swings: Hormonal variances can prompt changes in temperament, including crabbiness, nervousness, and wretchedness. Actual Changes: Numerous ladies experience weight gain, especially around the midsection, as well as diminishing hair and dry skin. Understanding these side effects and their effects can assist you with creating methodologies to oversee them. Every lady's involvement in menopause is novel, and side effects can shift broadly regarding type and seriousness. Meaning of Figuring out Menopause Understanding menopause is pivotal in light of multiple factors. In the first place, it enables you with the information expected to successfully perceive and oversee side effects. Rather than feeling overpowered or terrified by the progressions occurring in your body, you can move toward them with certainty and proactive procedures. Second, being educated about menopause can assist you with pursuing better wellbeing choices. Knowing what's in store permits you to plan for the change and look for suitable clinical counsel and medicines when vital. This can altogether work on your personal satisfaction during and after menopause.

Finally, understanding menopause can foster better communication with healthcare providers, partners, and support networks. By sharing your experiences and knowledge, you can build a supportive community that understands and respects your journey.

Conclusion Menopause is a huge life change that denotes the finish of contraceptive years and the start of another period of life. By grasping the definition, stages, and normal side effects of menopause, you can explore this excursion effortlessly and certainty. Information is power, and being educated about menopause is the most important move toward dealing with its difficulties and embracing the open doors it brings. In the accompanying sections, we will dive further into the particular parts of menopause, giving reasonable guidance and techniques to assist you with overseeing side effects and keep up with your general prosperity. Together, we will investigate the regular ways to deal with side effects of the executives, clinical medicines, mental and profound prosperity, sexual wellbeing, long haul wellbeing contemplations, and way of life changes. Welcome to the following part of your life — we should make it a solid, lively, and enabled one.

Chapter 2:

Early Signs and Symptoms

Menopause doesn't work out coincidentally; a slow change starts with perimenopause and advances to postmenopause. Perceiving the early signs and side effects can help you plan and deal with this huge life altering event all the more successfully. In this section, we will investigate the normal early side effects of menopause, their causes, and pragmatic ways to oversee them. Hot Blazes and Night Sweats Hot glimmers are one of the most notable side effects of menopause. They are unexpected, serious sensations of intensity that can spread all through your body, frequently joined by perspiring and a fast heartbeat. Night sweats are hot blazes that happen during rest, causing critical distress and disturbing rest. Causes: Hot blazes and night sweats are accepted to be brought about by changes in the body's indoor regulator, which is managed by the nerve center in light of fluctuating chemical levels, especially estrogen. The board

Tips: Keep Cool: Dress in layers and utilize a fan or cooling to remain cool. Keep away from Triggers: Normal triggers incorporate hot beverages, fiery food varieties, caffeine, and liquor. Distinguishing and keeping away from your own triggers can lessen the recurrence of hot blazes. Practice Unwinding Strategies: Profound breathing, reflection, and yoga can assist with overseeing pressure and lessen the seriousness of hot glimmers. Sporadic Periods One of the earliest indications of perimenopause is an adjustment of feminine cycle designs. You could see that your periods become more limited or longer, heavier or lighter, or more scattered. Causes: These progressions are because of the unpredictable arrival of eggs by the ovaries as chemical levels vacillate. The executives Tips: Track Your Cycle: Keeping a journal of your period can assist you with seeing themes and changes. Counsel Your Primary care physician: Assuming you experience very weighty draining or periods that last over about fourteen days, search clinical guidance to preclude different circumstances.

Rest Aggravations.

Numerous ladies experience trouble resting during perimenopause and menopause. This can incorporate difficulty nodding off, awakening often during the evening, or getting up too soon. Causes: Hormonal changes, night sweats, and expanded tension can all add to rest aggravations. **The executives Tips: Establish a Climate:** Guarantee your room is cool, dull, and calm that welcomes rests. Use power outage draperies and background noise if fundamental. Foster a Daily practice: Hit the sack and wake up simultaneously consistently, and lay out a quieting sleep time routine to indicate to your body that now is the ideal time to rest. **Stay away from Energizers:** Cutoff caffeine and liquor admission, particularly in the hours paving the way to sleep time. Temperament Swings and Close to home Changes Mind-set swings, crabbiness, and sensations of despondency or tension are normal during the menopausal process. These profound changes can be troubling and may influence your connections and day to day existence. **Causes**: Fluctuating chemical levels can influence synapses in the mind, prompting changes in temperament. **The executives Tips**: Work-out Routinely: Actual work can help your state of mind and diminish pressure. **Look for Help:** Conversing with companions, joining support gatherings, or looking for proficient directing can offer close to home help and commonsense exhortation. **Practice Care:** Methods like contemplation, profound breathing activities, and yoga can assist with overseeing pressure and work on close to home prosperity. Actual Changes Menopause can achieve different actual changes, including weight gain, diminishing hair, and dry skin. Causes: The reduction in estrogen levels influences digestion, skin versatility, and hair development. **The board Tips: Eat a Decent Eating routine**: Spotlight on a careful nutritional plan wealthy in organic products, vegetables, entire grains, and lean proteins to help generally wellbeing and oversee weight.

Remain Hydrated: Drinking a lot of water can assist with keeping up with skin hydration and flexibility. **Utilize Delicate Items**: Settle on delicate, saturating shampoos and skincare items to address hair and skin changes. Memory and Focus Issues A few ladies report encountering memory failures or trouble concentrating during menopause. These mental changes can be baffling and may influence day to day working. **Causes:** Hormonal changes, stress, and rest aggravations can all add to mental issues. **The board Tips: Remain Coordinated**: Use records, organizers, and suggestions to assist with monitoring undertakings and arrangements.

Remain Intellectually Dynamic: Participate in exercises that animate your cerebrum, like perusing, riddles, and mastering new abilities. **Deal with Your General Wellbeing**: Standard activity, a solid eating routine, and sufficient rest can all help mental capability. Conclusion: Perceiving and understanding the early signs and side effects of menopause is the most important move toward dealing with this progress with certainty. While these side effects can be challenging, there are numerous procedures and medicines accessible to assist you with adapting really. In the accompanying sections, we will investigate more meticulously the different ways to deal with overseeing menopause side effects, from regular solutions for clinical medicines. By outfitting yourself with information and viable instruments, you can explore this excursion with versatility and elegance. Keep in mind, you are in good company in this insight, and backing is dependably accessible. Together, we will investigate the ways to a better and more engaged life during and after menopause.

Chapter 3:

Hormonal Changes

Menopause is basically determined by hormonal changes that altogether influence your body and psyche. Understanding these hormonal movements can demystify a significant number of the side effects you experience and assist you with finding proactive ways to oversee them. In this section, we will investigate the jobs of estrogen and progesterone, the impacts of their variances, and the drawn out wellbeing ramifications of these changes. Estrogen and Progesterone: Key Chemicals Estrogen and progesterone are the essential chemicals associated with the feminine cycle and regenerative framework. They are delivered by the ovaries and assume significant parts in different physical processes: Estrogen: This chemical directs the period, keeps up with bone thickness, upholds cardiovascular wellbeing, and influences the cerebrum, skin, and urinary parcel. Progesterone: Fundamentally associated with setting up the body for pregnancy, progesterone likewise directs the feminine cycle and backing the coating of the uterus. As you approach menopause, the development of these chemicals starts to decline, prompting different physical and profound changes. Chemical Changes During Perimenopause Perimenopause, the temporary stage paving the way to menopause, is set apart by huge changes in chemical levels. During this time, the ovaries become less receptive to hormonal signs from the cerebrum, bringing about sporadic and capricious patterns of estrogen and progesterone. Estrogen: Levels might fluctuate generally, prompting side effects like hot blazes, night sweats, and emotional episodes. Elevated degrees of estrogen can cause side effects like delicate bosoms and swelling, while low levels can prompt vaginal dryness and diminished charisma. Progesterone: The decrease in progesterone frequently goes before the drop in estrogen, adding to unpredictable monthly cycles and expanded hazard of endometrial hyperplasia (thickening of the uterine covering). Influence on the Body: The vacillations and possible decrease in estrogen and progesterone levels influence numerous frameworks in the body, prompting a large number of side effects. Conceptual Framework: Sporadic periods and possible discontinuance of monthly cycle are the clearest signs. Diminished estrogen can likewise prompt vaginal dryness, diminishing of the vaginal walls, and decreased flexibility, which might cause distress during intercourse. Skeletal Framework: Estrogen keeps up with bone thickness. As levels decline, ladies are at expanded risk for osteoporosis, a condition where bones become feeble and weak. Cardiovascular Framework: Estrogen defensively affects the heart and veins. Lower levels can expand the gamble of cardiovascular illnesses, including coronary episode and stroke. Urinary Framework: Diminished estrogen can debilitate the tissues of the urinary plot, prompting side effects

like urinary incontinence and expanded chance of urinary parcel diseases (UTIs). Skin and Hair: Diminished estrogen can prompt diminishing skin, diminished collagen creation, and going bald. Mental Capability: Hormonal changes can influence synapses in the mind, prompting memory slips, trouble concentrating, and temperament swings.
Long haul Wellbeing Suggestions

Understanding the drawn out wellbeing ramifications of hormonal changes during menopause is vital for proactive administration and keeping up with in general wellbeing and prosperity: Bone Wellbeing: To battle the gamble of osteoporosis, guarantee sufficient admission of calcium and vitamin D, participate in weight-bearing activities, and think about meds whenever endorsed by your medical care supplier. Heart Wellbeing: Embrace a heart-solid way of life by keeping a decent eating routine, practicing consistently, and abstaining from smoking and exorbitant liquor utilization. Customary check-ups with your medical services supplier can assist with observing your cardiovascular wellbeing. Emotional wellness: Hormonal changes can influence psychological well-being, making it essential to address any side effects of nervousness, melancholy, or mental hardships. Remain intellectually dynamic, look for social help, and think about advising or prescription if vital. Adjusting Hormonal Changes There are different methodologies to assist with adjusting hormonal changes and reduce menopausal side effects: Chemical Substitution Treatment (HRT): HRT can actually lighten side effects by supplanting the chemicals your body does not create anymore. It is accessible in different structures, including pills, fixes, gels, and creams. Talk about the advantages and dangers of HRT with your medical care supplier to decide whether it is appropriate for you. Normal Cures: A few ladies find help through regular cures, for example, phytoestrogens (plant-based estrogens found in food sources like soy), dark cohosh, and red clover. Continuously counsel your medical services supplier prior to beginning any new enhancement. Way of life Changes: Taking on a sound way of life can assist with overseeing side effects. This remembers eating a fair eating routine rich in natural products, vegetables, and entire grains, practicing consistently, overseeing pressure through care or yoga, and getting sufficient rest. Conclusion Hormonal changes during menopause are a characteristic piece of maturing, however they can prompt various side effects and wellbeing gambles. By grasping the jobs of estrogen and progesterone, the impacts of their vacillations, and the drawn out wellbeing suggestions, you can find proactive ways to deal with these changes. Whether through chemical substitution treatment, normal cures, or way of life changes, there are numerous ways of adjusting these hormonal moves and keeping up with your wellbeing and prosperity. In the following part, we will investigate normal ways to deal with overseeing menopause side effects, giving commonsense guidance and methodologies to assist you explore this progress no sweat.

Chapter 4:

Managing Symptoms Naturally

Menopause is a tremendous life progress, and managing its secondary effects can be challenging. While clinical prescriptions like Hormone Replacement Treatment (HRT) are available, various women like to research customary ways of managing easing up their secondary effects. This part dives into various exhaustive systems, including diet, resolve, local fixes, and stress the leaders techniques, that can help you with investigating menopause, no perspiration and comfort. Diet and Food A fair eating routine is earnest for all things considered and can in a general sense impact menopausal secondary effects. The following are a couple of dietary frameworks to consider: Phytoestrogens: These plant-based intensifiers imitate estrogen in the body and can help with changing synthetic levels. Food assortments rich in phytoestrogens consolidate soy things (tofu, soy milk), flaxseeds, and vegetables. Calcium and Vitamin D: As estrogen levels drop, bone thickness can reduce, growing the risk of osteoporosis. Ensure adequate affirmation of calcium and vitamin D to assist with boning prosperity. Dairy things, blended greens, and propped food sources are incredible wellsprings of calcium, while sunshine and fortified food assortments can help you with getting adequate vitamin D. Strong Fats: Omega-3 unsaturated fats, found in fish, flaxseeds, and walnuts, can help with decreasing irritation and sponsorship heart prosperity. Verdant food varieties: An eating routine abundant in results of the dirt gives major supplements, minerals, and cell fortifications that assist by and large and help with administering weight. Hydration: Drinking a ton of water can help with regulating secondary effects like dry skin and vaginal dryness. Typical dynamic work offers different benefits for menopausal women, including secondary effects and general prosperity improvement: Weight The board: Exercise keeps a strong weight, which can reduce the risk of cardiovascular contaminations and diabetes. Bone Prosperity: Weight-bearing exercises, such as walking, running, and strength getting ready, help with staying aware of bone thickness and reduce the risk of osteoporosis. Close to home prosperity: Genuine work releases endorphins, which can additionally foster personality and lessening symptoms of pressure and hopelessness. Rest Quality: Common action can propel better rest by dealing with the rest wake cycle. Normal Fixes Various women go to regular answers for manage menopausal aftereffects. While these can be strong, it's basic to

chat with a clinical benefits provider preceding starting any new upgrade: Dim Cohosh: Often used to diminish hot glints and night sweats, dull cohosh is a well known local fix. In any case, its effects can change, and it may not be sensible for everyone. Red Clover: Contains phytoestrogens that can help with changing compound levels and straightforwardness hot bursts and night sweats. Dong Quai: Known as "female ginseng," dong quai is used in standard Chinese medicine to treat menopausal aftereffects, including hot gleams and ladylike abnormalities. Evening Primrose Oil: Affluent in gamma-linolenic destructive (GLA), evening primrose oil could help with decreasing chest delicacy and hormonal lopsided characters. Stress The board Procedures Stress can fuel menopausal side effects, making pressure the board vital for prosperity. Here are a few successful procedures:
Care and Contemplation: Rehearsing care and reflection can assist with lessening pressure, further develop state of mind, and improve by and large profound prosperity. Indeed, even a couple of moments of everyday contemplation can have a huge effect. Yoga: Yoga consolidates actual stances, breathing activities, and reflection, offering an all encompassing way to deal with overseeing pressure and further developing adaptability, strength, and equilibrium. Profound Breathing

Activities: Basic profound breathing activities can assist with quieting the psyche and decrease the force of hot blazes and nervousness. Journaling: Expounding on your viewpoints and sentiments can be a restorative method for overseeing pressure and gaining understanding into your close to home state. Rest Cleanliness Great rest cleanliness practices can assist with further developing rest quality and diminish a sleeping disorder: Lay out a Daily schedule: Hit the sack and wake up simultaneously consistently to direct your rest wake cycle. Establish a Loosening up Climate: Guarantee your room is cool, dim, and calm. Consider utilizing power outage shades, earplugs, or repetitive sound. Limit Screen Time: Stay away from screens (television, PC, cell phone) basically an hour prior to sleep time, as the blue light can impede melatonin creation. Stay away from Energizers: Decrease caffeine and liquor consumption, particularly in the hours paving the way to sleep time. Needle therapy and Back rub Treatment Elective treatments like needle therapy and back rub can give alleviation from menopausal side effects: Needle therapy: This conventional Chinese medication method includes embedding meager needles into explicit focuses on the body. It can assist with diminishing hot glimmers, night sweats, and work on generally speaking prosperity. Knead Treatment: Normal back rubs can assist with lessening pressure, further develop course, and ease muscle strain. Overseeing menopausal side effects normally includes a comprehensive methodology that incorporates diet, work out, home grown cures, stress the board, and elective treatments. These techniques can assist with easing side effects and work on your general personal satisfaction. Keep in mind, it's fundamental to talk with medical care experts prior to beginning any new therapies or enhancements to guarantee they are protected and proper for your singular necessities.

In the next chapter, we will explore medical treatments for menopause, including Hormone Replacement Therapy (HRT) and other pharmaceutical options. By understanding all available options, you can make informed decisions about how to best manage your menopause journey.

Chapter 5:

Medical Treatments for Menopause

While normal methodologies can altogether mitigate menopausal side effects, a few ladies might require or favor clinical medicines to really deal with their side effects. This part investigates different clinical therapies for menopause, including Chemical Substitution Treatment (CST), non-hormonal drugs, and other clinical mediations. Understanding these choices can assist you with coming to informed conclusions about your wellbeing and prosperity. Chemical Substitution Treatment (CST) Chemical Substitution Treatment is one of the best medicines for alleviating menopausal side effects. HRT includes the organization of estrogen or a blend of estrogen and progesterone to supplant the chemicals that the body does not create anymore. Kinds of CST: Estrogen Treatment (ET): Utilized basically for ladies who have had a hysterectomy. It includes taking estrogen alone. Consolidated Estrogen-Progestogen Treatment (EPT): For ladies with an unblemished uterus, a blend of estrogen and progesterone is recommended to forestall endometrial hyperplasia (thickening of the uterine covering). **Types**

 Pills: Oral tablets taken day to day. Patches: Applied to the skin and changed routinely. Gels and Creams: Applied to the skin and assimilated into the circulation system. Vaginal Rings, Tablets, and Creams: Used to lighten vaginal and urinary side effects by conveying estrogen straightforwardly to the vaginal tissues. Benefits: Alleviation from hot glimmers and night sweats. Further developed rest quality. Easing of vaginal dryness and uneasiness during intercourse. Counteraction of bone misfortune and decrease of break risk. Risks: Expanded hazard of blood clusters, stroke, and particular sorts of malignant growth (e.g., bosom disease) with long haul use. Potential aftereffects, for example, bulging, bosom delicacy, and state of mind changes. It's essential to examine the advantages and dangers of CST with your medical care supplier to decide the best game-plan in view of your singular wellbeing profile and side effects.

Non-Hormonal Prescriptions For ladies who can't or decide not to utilize HRT, a few non-hormonal prescriptions can assist with overseeing menopausal side effects: Specific Serotonin Reuptake Inhibitors (SSRIs) and Selective Norepinephrine

Reuptake Inhibitors (SNRIs): Initially used to treat discouragement and uneasiness, these meds can likewise decrease the recurrence and seriousness of hot blazes and night sweats. Models incorporate venlafaxine (Effexor), paroxetine (Paxil), and fluoxetine (Prozac). Gabapentin: An anticonvulsant drug that can assist with lessening hot glimmers, particularly around evening time. Clonidine: A circulatory strain drug that can assist with lessening hot glimmers and night sweats. Ospemifene (Osphena): A non-hormonal medicine used to treat vaginal dryness and difficult intercourse by copying the impacts of estrogen on vaginal tissues. Vaginal Estrogen For ladies encountering vaginal dryness, inconvenience during intercourse, or urinary side effects, confined vaginal estrogen treatment can be profoundly compelling: Structures: Creams, tablets, and rings that convey low portions of estrogen straightforwardly to the vaginal tissues. Benefits: Worked on vaginal oil, flexibility, and pH balance, which can lessen side effects like dryness, tingling, and agony during intercourse. Wellbeing: Vaginal estrogen is by and large viewed as protected with insignificant foundational retention, making it a reasonable choice for ladies who can't take fundamental HRT. **Bioidentical Chemical Treatment** Bioidentical chemicals are artificially indistinguishable from those the human body produces. They are accessible in FDA-supported structures and specially intensified arrangements: FDA-Endorsed Bioidentical Chemicals: These incorporate choices like estradiol and progesterone that are accessible in standard dosages and structures (e.g., patches, gels, pills). **Intensified Bioidentical Chemicals:** Exclusively blended by drug specialists as per a medical services supplier's remedy, custom-made to individual necessities. Nonetheless, intensified chemicals are not FDA-directed and may convey extra dangers connected with virtue and measurement consistency. Elective Clinical Medicines For ladies searching for elective clinical medicines, the accompanying choices might be thought of: Needle therapy: A few investigations propose that needle therapy can assist with decreasing the recurrence and seriousness of hot glimmers. Cognitive Behavioral Treatment (CBT): A kind of psychotherapy that can assist with overseeing emotional episodes, uneasiness, and rest unsettling influences by changing thought processes and conduct. Home grown Enhancements: While not stringently clinical, a few ladies find help with natural enhancements like dark cohosh, red clover, and night primrose oil. Notwithstanding, it is fundamental to examine these with a medical services supplier to guarantee security and viability. End Clinical medications for menopause offer an extent of decisions to direct incidental effects, as a matter of fact and work on private fulfillment. From HRT and non-hormonal drugs to restricted prescriptions and elective medicines, there are deals to fit various necessities and tendencies. It's vital to work personally with your clinical consideration provider to conclude the most fitting treatment plan considering your secondary effects, prosperity history, and individual tendencies. In the accompanying part, we will focus on mental and near and dear success during menopause, researching procedures to keep an elevating point of view and manage the individual challenges that much of the time go with this life change. Understanding and keeping an eye on the mental and near and dear pieces of menopause is fundamental to investigating this period with adaptability and ease.

Chapter 6:

Mental and Emotional Well-Being

Menopause brings actual changes as well as influences mental and profound wellbeing. This section dives into understanding these close to home moves and offers techniques to keep up with mental prosperity during this progress. Figuring out Close to home Changes Hormonal Impact on Mind-set: What estrogen and progesterone mean for cerebrum science and temperament. Normal Close to home Side effects: Emotional episodes, uneasiness, discouragement, crabbiness, and memory slips. Influence on Day to day existence: What close to home changes can mean for connections, work, and confidence. Ways of dealing with hardship or stress Care and Contemplation: Methods to remain present and lessen pressure. Cognitive Behavioral Treatment (CBT): How CBT can help reexamine negative contemplations and oversee nervousness and melancholy. Encouraging groups of people: The significance of social help from companions, family, and care groups. Solid Way of life Practices Actual work: How exercise benefits emotional wellness and lifts temperament. Nourishment: Food varieties that help cerebrum wellbeing and profound solidness. Rest Cleanliness: Methods for further developing rest quality to upgrade mental prosperity. Proficient Assistance When to Look for Help: Recognizing when close to home side effects require proficient mediation. Sorts of Treatment: Outline of various restorative methodologies, including psychotherapy, advising, and bunch treatment. Prescription Choices: Antidepressants, against nervousness drugs, and other pharmacological medicines for serious side effects. Taking care of oneself and Unwinding Methods Journaling: Involving composing as a device to handle feelings and lessen pressure. Imaginative Outlets: The job of leisure activities and innovative exercises in keeping up with emotional wellness. Unwinding Procedures: Profound breathing activities, yoga, and other unwinding rehearsals. Building Versatility Positive Reasoning: Developing an uplifting perspective and tracking down bliss in day to day existence. Objective Setting: Laying out reasonable objectives to keep up with inspiration and a feeling of direction. Adjusting to Change: Embracing the progressions that accompany menopause and tracking down new open doors for development. Connections and Correspondence Conveying Needs: Compelling correspondence with accomplices, family, and companions about profound requirements and encounters. Closeness and Association: Keeping up with closeness and association in connections during menopause. Managing Struggle: Techniques for overseeing clashes that emerge from profound changes. Strengthening and Self-Revelation Rediscovering Self: Involving menopause as a period for self-disclosure and strengthening. New Open doors: Investigating new interests, leisure activities, and vocation valuable open doors. Self-awareness: Embracing self-improvement and tracking down new reasons during this phase of life . Conclusion Keeping up with mental and close to home prosperity during menopause is critical for a solid and satisfying life. By understanding the close to home changes that go with this progress and utilizing powerful survival methods, you can explore this period with strength and inspiration. In the accompanying section, we will investigate the job of connections and closeness during menopause, giving experiences and tips to keeping up serious areas of strength for with, associations.

Chapter 7:

Relationships and Intimacy

Menopause can achieve tremendous changes in connections and closeness. Understanding these progressions and figuring out how to explore them can assist with keeping up areas of strength for with, associations with your accomplice, family, and companions. In this section, we will investigate the effect of menopause on connections, offer procedures to upgrade closeness, and give tips to powerful correspondence. **Grasping the Effect on Connections Close to Home Changes**: How emotional episodes, tension, and sadness can influence connections. **Actual Changes**: The effect of side effects like vaginal dryness, diminished moxie, and weakness on closeness. **Changes in Jobs**: Changes in relational peculiarities and jobs during menopause. **Improving Closeness Open Correspondence**: The significance of examining changes and needs with your accomplice. **Actual Warmth**: Keeping up with actual closeness through touch, embraces, and kisses. **Closeness Past Sex**: Investigating different types of closeness, like profound and scholarly associations. **Overseeing Actual Side effects Vaginal Ointments and Lotions:** Items to lighten vaginal dryness and distress during intercourse. **Pelvic Floor Activities:** Fortifying pelvic muscles to work on sexual capability and diminish urinary side effects. **Solid Way of life**: The job of diet, exercise, and hydration in upgrading sexual wellbeing. Profound Association Building **Trust and Understanding**: How compassion and support can reinforce your relationship. **Quality Time:** Setting aside a few minutes for shared exercises and encounters. Common Help: Supporting each other through individual and shared difficulties. **Tending to Sexual Well Being**

Sexual Wellbeing Training: Figuring out changes in sexual wellbeing and investigating arrangements.

Proficient Assistance: Looking for counsel from medical services suppliers or sex advisors if necessary. Trial and error and Investigation: Attempting new things to keep the sexual relationship energizing and satisfying. Reinforcing Family Connections Correspondence with Kids: Clarifying menopause for youngsters and keeping up with open lines of correspondence. More distant family Elements: Exploring changes in associations with more distant family individuals. Encouraging groups of people: Building and keeping major areas of strength for an organization of loved ones. Social Associations Companionship and Social Help: The significance of keeping up with and supporting fellowships. Local area Association: Taking part in local area exercises and tracking down new gatherings. Online People group: The advantages of joining on the web support gatherings and discussions for shared encounters and guidance.

Self-Disclosure and Self-improvement Investigating New Interests: Finding new leisure activities and exercises that give pleasure and satisfaction. Individual Objectives: Defining and accomplishing individual objectives to upgrade confidence and prosperity. Strengthening: Embracing this phase of life as a chance for development and self-disclosure. Conclusion Menopause can be a difficult time for connections and closeness, yet with open correspondence, understanding, and an eagerness to adjust, you can keep up with and even reinforce your associations. By tending to physical and close to home changes together, investigating better approaches to associate, and looking for help when required, you can explore this progress with certainty and love.

Chapter 8:

Self-Care and Lifestyle Changes

Menopause is a period of huge change, and dealing with yourself is a higher priority than at any other time. Carrying out taking care of oneself practices and making way of life changes can assist you with overseeing side effects, further develop your general prosperity, and explore this progress with certainty. In this section, we will investigate different ways of taking care of oneself and ways of life that can improve your personal satisfaction during menopause. Significance of Taking care of oneself Focusing on Yourself: Figuring out the significance of investing your necessities first and taking energy for taking care of oneself. All encompassing Methodology: Tending to physical, close to home, and emotional wellness through far reaching taking care of oneself practices. Nourishment and Diet Adjusted Diet: The job of a fair eating routine in overseeing menopausal side effects and supporting generally speaking wellbeing. Key Supplements: Fundamental supplements for menopausal ladies, including calcium, vitamin D, magnesium, and omega-3 unsaturated fats.

Good dieting Propensities: Ways to keep a solid eating regimen, for example, dinner arranging, segment control, and careful eating. Actual work Practice Advantages: How standard actual work can assist with overseeing weight, further develop mind-set, and diminish the gamble of constant illnesses. Sorts of Activity: Suggested practices for menopausal ladies, including cardio, strength preparing, adaptability activities, and equilibrium preparing. Making a Daily schedule: Fostering a predictable work-out schedule that accommodates your way of life and inclinations. Rest Cleanliness Rest Difficulties: Normal rest unsettling influences during menopause, for example, sleep deprivation and night sweats. Further developing Rest Quality: Methodologies for better rest, including keeping a standard rest plan, making a loosening up sleep time schedule, and streamlining your rest climate. Unwinding Procedures: Integrating unwinding strategies, like profound breathing, moderate muscle unwinding, and directed symbolism, to further develop rest quality. Stress The executives Effect of Pressure: What stress can fuel menopausal side effects and mean for in general wellbeing. Stress Decrease Procedures: Viable pressure on the executives methods, like care contemplation, yoga, and kendo. Using time effectively: Ways to deal with your time successfully to diminish pressure and make a healthy lifestyle. Psychological well-being Close to home Prosperity: Understanding the profound changes that accompany menopause and how to oversee them. Emotionally supportive networks: The significance of building and keeping up areas of strength with frameworks, including companions, family, and care groups. Proficient Assistance: When to look for proficient assistance from advisors or guides for close to home and emotional well-being support. Skin and Hair Care.

Skin Changes: Tending to normal skin changes during menopause, like dryness, diminishing, and expanded responsiveness. Skincare Schedule: Fostering a skincare schedule that incorporates delicate purifying, saturating, and sun insurance. Hair Care: Ways to oversee changes in hair surface and thickness, including the utilization of delicate hair care items and ordinary trims. Preventive Medical care Ordinary Check-Ups: The significance of normal clinical check-ups and screenings to screen your wellbeing. Vaccinations and Screenings: Keeping awake to-date with suggested immunizations and wellbeing screenings, for example, mammograms, bone thickness tests, and cholesterol checks. Solid Way of life Decisions: Pursuing way of life decisions that help long haul wellbeing, for example, abstaining from smoking, restricting liquor consumption, and keeping a sound weight. Self-improvement and Advancement Investigating New Interests: Utilizing this chance to investigate new side interests, interests, and exercises that give pleasure and satisfaction. Putting forth Objectives: Laying out private objectives and making an arrangement to accomplish them, encouraging a feeling of direction and achievement. Long lasting Picking up: Embracing open doors for deep rooted learning and self-improvement, like taking classes, going to studios, or acquiring new abilities. Conclusion Taking care of oneself and way of life changes are pivotal for overseeing menopausal side effects and keeping up with generally speaking prosperity. By focusing on your wellbeing, taking on a fair eating routine, remaining genuinely dynamic, overseeing pressure, and looking for help, you can explore menopause with versatility and certainty. Embrace this season of progress as a potential chance to zero in on yourself, investigate new interests, and develop a satisfying and sound life.

Chapter 9:

Financial Planning and Retirement Strategies

As you explore menopause and the changes it brings, getting your monetary future turns out to be progressively significant. Compelling monetary preparation and retirement procedures can give true serenity and guarantee you partake in an agreeable and stable future. In this section, we will investigate different parts of monetary preparation, including planning, saving, money management, and getting ready for retirement. Figuring out Monetary Necessities Surveying What is happening: Considering your pay, costs, obligations, and resources. Laying out Monetary Objectives: Characterizing present moment and long haul monetary objectives, like putting something aside for retirement, taking care of obligation, or financing significant buys. Making a Spending plan: Fostering a practical spending plan that lines up with your monetary objectives and way of life. Putting something aside for Retirement Retirement Records: Understanding various sorts of retirement accounts, for example, 401(k)s, IRAs, and Roth IRAs. Manager Supported Plans: Augmenting commitments to boss supported retirement plans and exploiting any matching commitments. Individual Reserve funds: Building individual investment funds through normal commitments to retirement accounts and different investment funds vehicles. Contributing Astutely Venture Rudiments: Grasping the standards of effective money management, including risk resilience, resource distribution, and enhancement. Sorts of Speculations: Investigating different venture choices, like stocks, securities, common assets, and land. Working with Monetary Consultants: The advantages of looking for proficient counsel and picking a trustworthy monetary guide to direct your speculation choices. Overseeing Obligation Obligation Appraisal: Assessing your ongoing obligation, including charge card adjusts, home loans, and credits. Obligation Decrease Methodologies: Fostering an arrangement to pay off and oversee obligation, like focusing on exorbitant interest obligations and merging credits. FICO rating The board: Understanding the significance of keeping a decent FICO assessment and how to further develop it. Medical care Arranging Health care coverage: Guaranteeing you have satisfactory health care coverage inclusion, particularly as you approach retirement age. Long haul Care Protection: Taking into account long haul care protection to cover potential future medical services needs. Wellbeing Bank accounts (HSAs): Using HSAs to put something aside for clinical costs and exploit tax breaks. Federal retirement aide and Benefits Grasping Federal retirement aide: Figuring out how Government backed retirement benefits work and deciding the best chance to begin gathering them. Benefits Plans: On the off chance that you have an annuity, understanding how it squeezes into your general retirement plan and what choices are accessible for getting benefits. Bequest Arranging Wills and Trusts: Making a will and, if proper, laying out trusts to guarantee your resources are disseminated by your desires. Legal authority: Assigning a confidant in person to pursue monetary and medical services choices for your benefit in the event that you become unfit to do as such. Recipient Assignments: Guaranteeing all recipient assignments on retirement accounts, insurance contracts, and different resources are state-of-the-art. Monetary Schooling and Assets Gotten the hang of: Remaining informed about monetary preparation through books, classes, online courses, and monetary news. Assets for Ladies: Using assets explicitly intended for ladies, for example, monetary arranging studios and care groups. Making arrangements for Delight Relaxation and Travel: Planning for recreation exercises and going to guarantee you partake in your retirement years. Leisure activities and Interests: Saving assets to seek after new leisure activities and interests that give pleasure and satisfaction. Charitable effort: Investigating open doors for humanitarian effort and local area association that can advance your retirement experience. Conclusion: Monetary preparation and retirement techniques are fundamental for guaranteeing a protected and satisfying future. By figuring out your monetary necessities, saving and contributing admirably, overseeing obligations, and making arrangements for medical care and home matters, you can explore menopause and the past with certainty. Assume command over your monetary wellbeing today to partake in a steady and prosperous retirement. In the following part, we will zero in on self-awareness and tracking down reason in life after menopause. Embracing this stage as a chance for development and self-disclosure can prompt a more significant and improved life.

Chapter 10:

Personal Development and Finding Purpose

Considering getting back to the everyday schedule postgraduate education or accreditations. Remaining Informed: Staying up with the latest with recent developments, patterns, and progressions in areas of interest. Chipping in and Local area Association Offering in return: Finding reason through charitable effort and local area administration. Building Associations: Framing significant associations with others through shared volunteer encounters. Effect and Heritage: Figuring out the effect of your commitments and making an enduring inheritance. Improving Individual Connections Developing Associations: Fortifying associations with family, companions, and accomplices through superior correspondence and compassion. Fabricating New Fellowships: Extending your group of friends by joining clubs, gatherings, or online networks. Emotionally supportive networks: Fostering a strong encouraging group of people to share encounters and get consolation. Encouraging Profound Development Investigating Otherworldliness: Diving into profound practices that impact you, like contemplation, petition, or care. Discovering a sense of reconciliation: Methods for discovering a sense of reconciliation and happiness during life changes. Profound People group: Drawing in with otherworldly or strict networks for help and shared encounters. Wellbeing and Health Actual Wellbeing: Focusing on actual wellbeing through normal activity, adjusted nourishment, and routine clinical consideration. Mental Wellbeing: Zeroing in on psychological well-being through care rehearses, stress the board, and looking for proficient assistance if necessary. All encompassing Methodologies: Consolidating comprehensive wellbeing rehearses, like yoga, needle therapy, or fragrant healing. Exploring Profession Changes Vocation Advancement: Investigating open doors for professional development, change, or business. Balance between fun and serious activities: Techniques for accomplishing a sound balance between serious and fun activities that upholds individual prosperity. Mentorship and Training: Looking for mentorship or instructing for vocation direction and backing. Developing Flexibility Building Flexibility: Creating versatility to explore the difficulties and changes of menopause and then some. Positive Outlook: Developing a positive mentality to move toward life's changes with confidence and strength. Self-Sympathy: Rehearsing self-empathy and thoughtfulness towards yourself during times of progress and development. Conclusion Menopause is a period of huge change, however it likewise offers a special chance for self-awareness and tracking down new reasons. By embracing change, defining new objectives, investigating interests, and encouraging connections, you can lead a satisfying and improved life. Utilize this stage as a springboard for development, self-revelation, and making a significant future.

Chapter 11:

Menopause Myths and Facts

Although menopause is a natural part of a woman's life, there are still many misconceptions and myths about it. These fantasies can make pointless apprehension and disarray, making it crucial for isolated reality from fiction. In this part, we will expose normal legends about menopause and give exact data to assist you explore this progress with certainty and understanding. Common Myths Busted Legend: Menopause Comes about more or less by accident Truth: Menopause is a steady cycle that happens more than quite a long while. It typically begins during the transitional period known as perimenopause, during which hormone levels fluctuate, resulting in symptoms and shifts in menstrual cycles. Before reaching menopause, which is defined as having no menstrual periods for 12 consecutive months, this phase can last several years. After menopause, ladies enter postmenopause, a stage that goes on until the end of their lives. Myth: Only older women experience menopause.Truth: While the typical time of menopause is around 51, it can happen prior or later. Before age 40, early menopause can occur as a result of health conditions, medical treatments, or genetics. Ladies as youthful as their 30s can encounter premenopausal side effects. It's essential to perceive that menopause can change broadly in its beginning and movement. Fantasy: All Ladies Experience Similar Side effects Reality: Menopause is a profoundly individual encounter. Some women may experience severe symptoms like night sweats, hot flashes, and mood swings, while others may experience mild or no symptoms at all. The severity and type of symptoms experienced are significantly influenced by genetics, lifestyle, and overall health. Legend: Menopause Closures Sexual Longing Reality: Menopause isn't guaranteed to end sexual craving. While hormonal changes can influence drive, numerous ladies keep on having a fantastic sexual coexistence during and after menopause. Factors like close to home closeness, by and large wellbeing, and relationship quality assume critical parts in keeping up with sexual longing. Tending to actual side effects like vaginal dryness with greases or clinical medicines can likewise work on sexual solace and pleasure. Figuring out Current realities

The fact is that menopause is a biological process. Clarification: Menopause denotes the finish of a lady's conception years. The gradual decline in ovarian function and hormone production, particularly estrogen and progesterone, is the cause of this natural process. Understanding this can assist ladies with moving toward menopause unafraid, seeing it as an ordinary phase of life. It is a fact that lifestyle choices can affect symptoms. Explanation: Making healthy lifestyle choices can have a big effect on how menopausal symptoms are treated and how severe they are. A healthy diet, regular exercise, getting enough sleep, and learning how to manage stress can all help reduce symptoms and improve well-being in general. Maintaining a healthy weight, limiting alcohol consumption, and avoiding smoking are also beneficial. Fact: Mental Health Can Be Affected by Menopause Clarification: Hormonal changes during menopause can impact mind science, influencing temperament and psychological wellness. Ladies might encounter uneasiness, sorrow, touchiness, and memory slips. Perceiving these progressions as a component of the menopausal change can assist in looking for with appropriating backing and treatment, whether through way of life changes, guiding, or drug. Getting Rid of Other Common Myths Fantasy: Hormone Replacement Therapy (HRT) Is

Hazardous for All Ladies Reality: HRT can be a protected and compelling treatment for some ladies, especially when begun near the beginning of menopause. It can reduce side effects, for example, hot blazes, night sweats, and vaginal dryness, and furthermore assist with forestalling bone misfortune. Nonetheless, it isn't reasonable for everybody, and the choice to utilize HRT ought to be made in discussion with a medical services supplier, taking into account individual wellbeing dangers and advantages. Fantasy: Menopause Implies the Finish of Efficiency Reality: Menopause doesn't check the finish of a lady's useful or dynamic life. This stage offers new opportunities for personal development, career advancement, and creativity, which many women find liberating. It's a good time to take care of yourself, look into new interests, and take on new roles. Myth: During menopause, weight gain is inevitable. Fact: Although hormonal changes can make it harder to control weight, weight gain is not always inevitable. A mix of smart dieting, normal active work, and way of life changes can assist with keeping a sound weight. Understanding and overseeing factors like digestion changes and bulk misfortune are critical to successfully weigh the executives. Advice on How to Get Through Menopause Learn for Yourself Read trustworthy sources of information about menopause to stay informed about what to expect and how to deal with symptoms. Consult Healthcare Professionals: Getting regular checkups and having conversations with healthcare professionals can help create a management plan that meets your requirements. Get into good habits. Adjusted Diet: Spotlight on supplement thick food sources that help generally wellbeing. Customary Activity: Integrate cardiovascular, strength preparing, and adaptability practices into your daily schedule. Stress The board: Practice care, reflection, and unwinding procedures to lessen pressure. Fabricate an Emotionally supportive network Look for Help: Join support gatherings or discussions where you can share encounters and gain bits of knowledge from others going through menopause. Openly discuss your experiences with family and friends to build support and understanding. Investigate Treatment Choices Treatments: If your symptoms are severe, you should think about HRT and medications that don't use hormones. Elective Treatments: Investigate correlative treatments like needle therapy, natural enhancements, and yoga to oversee side effects. Conclusion Understanding and exposing menopause legends is pivotal for a positive and informed insight. You can approach menopause with confidence and the knowledge to make informed decisions about your health and well-being by distinguishing fact from fiction. With the knowledge that you are supported by accurate information and useful strategies, view this stage as an opportunity for personal development and discovery.

Chapter 12:

Alternative and Complementary Therapies

Many women seek alternative and complementary therapies to manage their symptoms and improve their overall health as they go through menopause. Without relying solely on conventional medical treatments, these strategies can provide relief and enhance quality of life. In this part, we will investigate different elective treatments, including needle therapy, natural enhancements, homeopathy, and reciprocal practices like back rub treatment, fragrant healing, and psyche body methods. Investigating Other Treatment Options Acupuncture What is Needle therapy?: Needle therapy is a conventional Chinese medication practice that includes embedding slight needles into explicit focuses on the body to adjust the body's energy stream, or "qi." Benefits for Menopause: Needle therapy has been displayed to assist with lessening the recurrence and seriousness of hot blazes, night sweats, and uneasiness. It might likewise further develop rest and in general prosperity. What's in store: A run of the mill needle therapy meeting includes an exhaustive counsel followed by the inclusion of needles, which are left set up for around 20-30 minutes. Meetings are by and large unwinding and torment free. Home grown Enhancements Dark Cohosh: Known for its viability in diminishing hot glimmers and night sweats, dark cohosh is a famous decision among menopausal ladies. However, it should only be used under the supervision of a medical professional and with extreme caution. Red Clover: This spice contains phytoestrogens that can assist with adjusting chemical levels and mitigate side effects like hot glimmers and vaginal dryness. Dong Quai: Frequently alluded to as "female ginseng," dong quai is utilized in customary Chinese medication to treat menopausal side effects, including hot glimmers and emotional episodes. Evening Primrose Oil: Wealthy in gamma-linolenic corrosive (GLA), evening primrose oil might assist with lessening bosom delicacy and hormonal uneven characters. Homeopathy Standards of Homeopathy: Homeopathy depends on the guideline of "like fixes like," utilizing profoundly weakened substances to animate the body's normal recuperating processes. Normal Cures: Homeopathic cures like Sepia, Lachesis, and Sulfur are in many cases used to deal with menopausal side effects like hot glimmers, crabbiness, and weakness. Treatment and Consultation: A homeopath will consult with you in detail to determine the best course of action for your symptoms and overall health. Corresponding Practices The Art of Massage Benefits: Normal back rubs can assist with lessening pressure, ease muscle strain, and further develop dissemination. They can also help you relax and feel better in general. Kinds of Back rub: Different sorts of back rub, like Swedish, profound tissue, and fragrance based treatment rub, can be useful for menopausal ladies. What to Expect: During a massage, a skilled therapist will manipulate the muscles and soft tissues in a variety of ways to induce relaxation and alleviate pain. Aromatherapy What is aromatherapy? It is the use of plant-derived essential oils to improve health and well-being.

These oils can be used in baths, on the skin, or inhaled.
Benefits for Menopause: Medicinal ointments like lavender,
peppermint, and clary sage can assist with overseeing side
effects like hot glimmers, sleep deprivation, and uneasiness.
Utilizing Essential Oils: Essential oils can be infused into bath
water, diffused into the air, or combined with carrier oils for
topical use. Always use essential oils safely, and if you need
help, talk to a professional. Mind-Body Practices Yoga: To
improve flexibility, strength, and mental clarity, yoga
incorporates meditation, physical postures, and breathing
exercises. It can assist with lessening pressure, further develop
mind-set, and ease menopausal side effects. Tai Chi and
Qigong are ancient Chinese exercises that combine meditation,
controlled breathing, and slow, deliberate movements. They
can assist with further developing equilibrium, lessen pressure,
and improve in general prosperity. Contemplation and Care:
Rehearsing care and reflection can assist with overseeing
pressure, further develop center, and advance close to home
equilibrium. Methods like directed reflection, profound
breathing activities, and care practices can be effectively
integrated into everyday schedules. Integrating
Complementary and Alternative Therapies Talking with
Medical care Suppliers To ensure a holistic and coordinated

approach to managing menopausal symptoms, discuss your interest in alternative and complementary therapies with your healthcare provider. Security and Viability: Guarantee that any elective treatments you pick are protected and compelling for your particular wellbeing needs and conditions. Keep away from self-endorsing and look for proficient direction. Making a Customized Plan Individualized Care: To address your unique symptoms and health objectives, create an individualized care plan that incorporates a combination of conventional and alternative treatments. Observing Advancement: Routinely survey the viability of the treatments you are involving and make changes depending on the situation. Monitor any progressions in side effects and by and large prosperity. Conclusion The management of menopausal symptoms and the improvement of one's overall well-being are both made possible by complementary and alternative treatments. By investigating approaches like needle therapy, natural enhancements, homeopathy, knead treatment, fragrant healing, and psyche body rehearses, you can make a complete and customized plan to explore menopause effortlessly and solace. Make sure to talk with medical services experts to guarantee the wellbeing and viability of these treatments and to coordinate them really into your general wellbeing routine.

Chapter 13:

Managing Chronic Conditions During Menopause

Menopause can introduce special difficulties for ladies who are likewise overseeing constant medical issues. The treatment of these conditions can be affected by the hormonal changes and symptoms of menopause. In this section, we will investigate techniques for overseeing normal ongoing circumstances during menopause, including diabetes, coronary illness, and osteoporosis. We will likewise talk about the significance of working intimately with medical services suppliers to guarantee complete and facilitated care. Figuring out the Interaction Among Menopause and Constant Circumstances Hormonal Impact: How chronic conditions are affected by the decline in estrogen and progesterone. Symptom Overlap: identifying symptoms like fatigue, weight gain, and changes in mood that could be brought on by both menopause and chronic conditions. The importance of proactive management and the fact that menopause can raise the risk of certain chronic conditions are two risk factors. Diabetes Management During Menopause Glucose Control Understanding how hormonal changes can affect insulin sensitivity and blood sugar levels is called hormonal fluctuations. Observing: Ordinary glucose checking to distinguish designs and change treatment designs as needs be. Diet and exercise: Managing blood sugar levels requires a well-balanced diet and regular exercise. Control of Medication Changing Drugs: Working with medical care suppliers to change diabetes prescriptions on a case by case basis during menopause. New Medicines: Investigating new meds or treatment choices that might be more viable during this phase of life. Choices for a Healthy Lifestyle Nourishment: Stressing an eating regimen wealthy in fiber, lean proteins, and sound fats to assist with overseeing glucose levels. Actual work: Integrating both cardiovascular and strength preparing activities to further develop insulin responsiveness and in general wellbeing. Stress The board: Utilizing procedures like care, contemplation, and yoga to decrease pressure, which can affect glucose control. Overseeing Coronary illness During Menopause Condition of the Heart Increased Danger: Recognizing how the loss of estrogen raises the risk of cardiovascular disease and stroke. Customary Screenings: Significance of ordinary check-ups and cardiovascular screenings, including circulatory strain, cholesterol, and fatty oil levels. Side effect Mindfulness:

Perceiving side effects of coronary illness, for example, chest torment, windedness, and surprising weakness. Solid Heart Propensities Diet: Emphasis on a heart-healthy diet full of whole grains, fruits, and vegetables. Work out: Integrating standard active work, including vigorous activities and strength preparing, to work on cardiovascular wellbeing. Smoking Suspension: Significance of stopping smoking to lessen the gamble of coronary illness and other medical problems. Prescription and Treatment Prescriptions: Working with medical care suppliers to oversee meds for pulse, cholesterol, and other heart-related conditions. Lifestyle Changes: Changing one's lifestyle to support heart health, such as limiting alcohol consumption, managing one's weight, and consuming less sodium. How to Treat Osteoporosis After Menopause Bone Wellbeing Effect of Estrogen Decline: Understanding how the decrease in estrogen during menopause speeds up bone misfortune. Risk Variables: Recognizing risk factors for osteoporosis, like family ancestry, smoking, and exorbitant liquor utilization. Preventive Measures Calcium and Vitamin D: Guaranteeing sufficient admission of calcium and vitamin D through diet and enhancements to help bone wellbeing. Weight-Bearing Activities: Consolidating weight-bearing and obstruction activities to fortify bones and diminish the gamble of cracks. Bone Thickness Testing: Customary bone thickness tests to screen bone wellbeing and identify early indications of osteoporosis. Treatment Choices Meds: Investigating meds that can assist with forestalling bone misfortune and reinforce bones, for example, bisphosphonates, particular estrogen receptor modulators (SERMs), and chemical substitution treatment (HRT). Lifestyle Changes: To support bone health, make changes to your lifestyle, like not drinking too much alcohol or smoking. Collaboration with Medical Professionals Facilitated Care Exhaustive Methodology: Significance of a complete and facilitated way to deal with overseeing menopause and persistent circumstances. Customary Check-Ups: Planning ordinary check-ups with medical care suppliers to screen wellbeing and change therapy plans on a case by case basis. Correspondence: Keeping up with transparent correspondence with medical services suppliers about side effects, therapies, and way of life changes. Plans for Individualized Treatment Customized Care: Creating individualized treatment designs that consider the extraordinary necessities and ailments of every lady. Taking a holistic approach to health management means taking into account both conventional and alternative treatments. Overseeing ongoing circumstances during menopause requires a proactive and complete methodology. By understanding the interaction among menopause and constant circumstances, ladies can do whatever it may take to keep up with their wellbeing and prosperity. Effective management necessitates regular checkups, healthy lifestyle choices, and close collaboration with healthcare providers. Embrace this phase of existence with certainty, realizing that you have the information and apparatuses to explore both menopause and persistent medical issues effectively.

Chapter 14:

Menopause in Different Cultures

Despite the fact that menopause is a universal experience, cultural perceptions and approaches to managing it can vary significantly. Understanding these assorted viewpoints can give significant bits of knowledge and elective ways to deal with overseeing menopause. In this section, we will investigate how different societies all over the planet view menopause, the conventional practices they use to oversee side effects, and what we can gain from these assorted methodologies. Social Perspectives Toward Menopause Western Societies Medicalization of Menopause: In numerous Western societies, menopause is many times seen through a clinical focal point, with an accentuation on side effects of the executives through chemical substitution treatment (HRT) and other clinical therapies. Cultural Stigma: Women's perceptions and experiences of menopause are influenced by the cultural stigma that arises when menopause is associated with aging and a loss of femininity. Asian Societies Menopause is regarded as a natural and positive life transition in many Asian cultures. Ayurveda and Traditional Chinese Medicine (TCM) often focus on balancing the energies in the body to manage symptoms. Regard for Seniors: Menopause is frequently connected with acquiring shrewdness and regard locally, as more seasoned ladies are adored for their experience and information. African Traditions Support from the Community: In a lot of African cultures, menopause is a communal experience with a lot of social support. Advice and support for women frequently come from traditional healers and community networks. Rituals and Traditions: This life stage is honored through a variety of rituals and traditions that help women get through the transition. Cultures of the Old World All encompassing Methodology: Native societies frequently adopt a comprehensive strategy to wellbeing, integrating otherworldly, physical, and close to home perspectives. The menopause is regarded as a time of change and renewal.

Utilization of Regular Cures: Conventional information on spices and normal cures is frequently used to oversee menopausal side effects. Conventional Practices and Cures Customary Chinese Medication (TCM) Home grown Medication: TCM utilizes different spices, for example, dong quai, ginseng, and dark cohosh, to adjust chemicals and reduce side effects. Needle therapy: Needle therapy is normally used to direct the body's energy stream and lessen side effects like hot glimmers and uneasiness. Dietary Treatment: Accentuation on a decent eating regimen rich in phytoestrogens, found in food varieties like soy, to help hormonal equilibrium. Ayurveda Dosha Balancing: Diet, lifestyle, and herbal remedies are all used in Ayurveda to bring the body's doshas (vata, pitta, and kapha) into balance. Rasayanas: These reviving spices and recipes, for example, ashwagandha and shatavari, are utilized to help essentialness and hormonal equilibrium. Panchakarma is a form of body cleansing and rejuvenation known as panchakarma. African Customary Medication Natural Cures: Utilization of native plants and spices, like red clover and sage, to oversee side effects. Otherworldly Practices: Fuse of profound practices and ceremonies to help close to home and actual prosperity. Local area Mending: Dependence on local area healers and encouraging groups of people for direction and backing. Practices of Native Americans Knowledge of herbs: Symptom management with native plants like black cohosh, sage, and wild yam. Participation in spiritual ceremonies and rituals to honor the transition and seek guidance from ancestors is known as spiritual ceremonies. All encompassing Wellbeing: Accentuation on keeping up with equilibrium and amiability inside the body, psyche, and soul. Illustrations from Worldwide Practices Implementing Effective Methods Comprehensive Methodologies: Embrace all encompassing methodologies that consider physical, profound, and otherworldly prosperity. Natural Remedies: Investigate the utilization of traditional herbs and natural remedies in conjunction with conventional treatments. Social Insight: Gain from the insight of various societies to make a more customized and socially delicate way to deal with overseeing menopause. Regarding Variety Social Awareness: Perceive and regard the assorted manners by which ladies experience and oversee menopause all over the planet. Inclusivity: Recognize that there is no one-size-fits-all approach and promote inclusivity and openness in discussions about menopause. Investigating menopause according to a worldwide viewpoint uncovers the rich variety of encounters and ways to deal with this life progress. By getting it and valuing these social distinctions, we can acquire new experiences and possibly integrate advantageous practices into our own lives. Embrace the insight of various societies and utilize this information to explore menopause with certainty, regard, and a feeling of association with ladies all over the planet. We will talk about how to keep work and menopause in balance.

Chapter 15:

Balancing Work and Menopause

Maintaining a successful career while going through menopause can be difficult, but it is possible to manage symptoms and thrive at work with the right strategies and support. This part gives reasonable counsel on overseeing menopausal side effects at work, speaking with managers, investigating profession changes, and accomplishing a sound balance between serious and fun activities. Workplace Symptom Management Hot Blazes and Night Sweats Dress in layers and keep a fan at your desk to keep cool. Pick breathable textures and think about keeping a difference in garments at work. Hydration: Consume a lot of water to keep hydrated and aid in temperature regulation. Cold Packs: During hot flashes, use cold packs or cooling towels in the office. Problems with sleep and fatigue Rest Breaks: Throughout the day, take regular, brief breaks to rest and recharge. A short walk or a few minutes of deep breathing can help. Rest Rooms: In the event that your work environment has a peaceful room or rest room, use it for a short reprieve during lunch or breaks. Solid Tidbits: Keep sound bites, like nuts and natural products, at your work area to keep up with energy levels. Changes in mood and emotions Stress The executives: Practice pressure the board strategies like care, reflection, and profound breathing activities. Proficient Assistance: Think about talking with an instructor or specialist in the event that close to home changes are affecting your work. Encouraging groups of people: Construct an encouraging group of people or partners who get it and can offer help when required. Mental Changes Tools for Organization: To stay on top of tasks, use tools for organization like planners, to-do lists, and digital reminders. Focus on Undertakings: Spotlight on high-need errands when you are generally ready and useful. Continuous Learning: Engage in activities like solving puzzles or learning new skills that stimulate your mind and improve cognitive function. Speaking with Bosses Open Exchange Start Discussions: In the event that you feel great, start a discussion with your boss or HR division about your menopause side effects and what they might mean for your work. Tell the truth: Speak the truth about your necessities and any facilities that could end up being useful to you to oversee side effects, like adaptable working hours or a cooler workplace. Mentioning Facilities Adaptable Hours: Solicitation adaptable working hours or the choice to telecommute if necessary to oversee side effects. Ecological Changes: Request changes like a fan at your work area, admittance to a peaceful room, or a more agreeable workstation. Lawful Privileges Know Your Privileges: Comprehend your legitimate freedoms with respect to working environment facilities and against segregation regulations in your country. Look for Help: If fundamental, look for help from working environment advocates or lawful experts to guarantee your freedoms are regarded. Vocation Advances and Valuable open doors Examining Brand-New Possibilities Profession Changes: Consider in the event that this phase of life is a great opportunity to investigate new vocation open doors or advances. Changing careers, pursuing a passion project, or starting your own business are all options for this. Further Education: If you want to improve your skills and discover new career paths, take advantage of opportunities for additional training or education. Entrepreneurship Beginning a Business: In the event that you have a business thought or purposeful venture, menopause may be the ideal opportunity to seek after business. Business Arranging: Foster a strong marketable strategy, look for mentorship, and exploit assets accessible for new business people. Coaching and Administration Mentorship Jobs: Think about taking on mentorship jobs to help more youthful associates and offer your experience and information. Leadership Possibilities:

Look into leadership positions within your company in order to put your knowledge and abilities to good use. Accomplishing Balance between serious and fun activities Defining Limits Work Hours: Put down clear stopping points for work hours and stick to them to guarantee you possess energy for rest and individual exercises. Separating: Put forth a cognizant attempt to detach from business related interchanges beyond working hours. Self-Care Schedule time for activities that promote well-being, such as exercise, hobbies, and relaxation, to make self-care a priority. Solid Way of life: Keep a sound way of life through adjusted sustenance, normal actual work, and satisfactory rest. Systems of Support Building Support: Establish a network of friends, family, and coworkers who can assist and comprehend. Proficient Help: Make it a point to proficient help, like guiding or training, to assist you with overseeing balance between serious and fun activities successfully. Conclusion: Adjusting work and menopause requires a proactive way to deal with overseeing side effects, powerful correspondence with bosses, and focusing on taking care of oneself. You can navigate this life transition while maintaining a successful and fulfilling career by implementing these strategies. Keep in mind that you are not the only woman facing similar difficulties; with the right resources and support, you can succeed both personally and professionally

. **Chapter 16:**

Personal Stories and Testimonials

Hearing from other people who have explored menopause can give important bits of knowledge, motivation, and a feeling of local area. Women whose experiences with menopause have been successful are profiled and praised in this chapter. These genuine encounters feature different viewpoints, survival techniques, and illustrations picked up, offering consolation and backing to those going through comparative changes. Individual Stories 1. Jane's Excursion: Embracing Change Background: In her late 40s, 52-year-old marketing executive Jane began to experience perimenopausal symptoms. Problems: She had trouble sleeping, hot flashes, and mood swings, which affected how well she did at work and in her personal life. Jane used holistic coping strategies like regular exercise, yoga, and a well-balanced diet high in phytoestrogens. She likewise rehearsed care reflection to oversee pressure and further develop rest. Results: Jane discovered that these changes to her lifestyle significantly reduced her symptoms. She likewise looked for help from a menopause support bunch, which helped her vibe less disconnected. Today, Jane feels engaged and more in charge of her wellbeing. 2. Maria's Story: How to Get Through Emotional Chaos Foundation: Maria, a 48-year-old instructor, battled with serious emotional episodes and uneasiness during perimenopause. Challenges: Her profound changes influenced her connections and made it hard to keep up with her typical inspirational perspective. Methods for dealing with especially difficult times: Maria looked for help from an advisor working in ladies' wellbeing and began cognitive Behavioral treatment (CBT). She also joined a nearby support group, where she could talk about her struggles and get support. Result: Through treatment and local area support, Maria figured out how to deal with her close to home side effects better. She presently feels more adjusted and can partake in her work and individual life once more. 3. Aisha's Story: Leveraging Community for Strength Foundation: Aisha, a 55-year-old local area coordinator, experienced menopause as a period of both physical and otherworldly change. Challenges: Aisha managed joint torment, weight gain, and night sweats, which upset her everyday practice. Survival techniques: She went to customary African cures and works on, including natural teas and profound ceremonies. Aisha also found strength in her community by taking part in activities for the community and women's circles. Result: Aisha's all encompassing and local area centered approach assisted her with dealing with her side effects and keeping an uplifting perspective. She feels a more profound association with her social legacy and a restored feeling of direction. 4. Lucy's Way: Adjusting Profession and Menopause Background: Lucy, a 50-year-old lawyer, struggled to balance her demanding career with menopause. Challenges: Hot blazes, exhaustion, and mind haze made it hard to keep up with her efficiency and certainty at work. Coping Strategies: Lucy openly discussed her symptoms with her employer, which resulted in more accommodating working hours and a more welcoming workplace. She likewise started utilizing natural enhancements and focused on ordinary activity. Result: With her manager's help and her proactive wellbeing measures, Lucy figured out how to keep up with her professional execution and further develop her general prosperity. She currently advocates for work environment approaches that help ladies going through menopause. 5. Mei's Understanding: The Job of Conventional Medication Foundation: Mei, a 53-year-old Artist, moved toward menopause with the information on Traditional Chinese Medicine (TCM). Challenges: She encountered extreme hot blazes and sleep deprivation, which impacted her imaginative work and day to day existence. Mei implemented acupuncture, herbal medicine, and dietary changes into her routine after consulting a TCM practitioner. Results: Mei was able to significantly reduce her symptoms as a result of these traditional practices. She found new inspiration in her art as she regained her creativity and vitality. Mei's experience affirmed her belief in the advantages of combining modern and traditional medicine. Expert Discussions Conversation with Dr. Specialist in Menopause, Sarah Thompson Foundation: Dr. Sarah Thompson is a prestigious menopause expert with more than 20 years of involvement with ladies' wellbeing. Key Bits of knowledge: Dr. Thompson emphasizes the benefits of both conventional and alternative treatments as well as the significance of individualized care. She features the requirement for ladies to advocate for them and search out the help and assets they need. Exhortation: "Each lady's menopause process is interesting. It's pivotal to pay attention to your body, remain informed, and not hold back to look for proficient assistance when required. A strong organization, whether it's family, companions, or a medical services group, can have a significant effect." Interview with Lisa Roberts, Mental Conduct Advisor Background: Lisa Roberts is a cognitive behavioral therapist who focuses on assisting women with emotional menopause management. Key Experiences: Lisa examines the normal personal difficulties ladies face during menopause and how CBT can help reexamine pessimistic contemplations and foster survival techniques. Guidance: "Don't misjudge the force of your brain in overseeing menopause. Tools for effectively managing stress, anxiety, and mood swings can be provided by CBT. It's tied in with building versatility and tracking down balance." What We've Learned Wisdom from All Tips for Managing Symptoms: Women share their practical advice, such as how to use cooling pillows, keep a menopause journal, and practice gratitude. Emotionally supportive networks: The significance of building major areas of strength for a framework is featured, whether through help gatherings, online networks, or dear loved ones. Self-Compassion: During this transition, many women emphasize the significance of self-compassion and patience. Well-being can be significantly improved by acknowledging that menopause is a natural phase and giving oneself time to adjust. Helpful Statements "Menopause isn't a closure; it's a fresh start loaded up with open doors for development and self-disclosure." - Jane "Through the highs and lows, I figured out how to pay attention to my body and give it the consideration it merits." - Maria "Finding strength in the local area and custom helped me embrace this change with elegance." - Aisha Lucy says,

"Balancing work and menopause can be accomplished with open communication and proactive measures." "Coordinating customary practices brought me harmony and restored my imaginative soul." - Mei. Conclusion Individual stories and tributes give significant viewpoints on exploring menopause. These genuine encounters feature the assorted ways ladies adapt to and beat the difficulties of this change. By sharing these accounts, we desire to move and support others on their menopause process, advising them that they are in good company and that there is strength in the local area and shared shrewdness.

Chapter 17

Final Reflection and Moving Forward

As "The Menopause Guide" comes to an end, it's time to look ahead with optimism and confidence and reflect on our journey together. This concluding chapter provides a summary of the most important takeaways, motivational insights, and suggestions for continuing to embrace this life-altering phase with strength and resilience. Taking Stock of the Journey: Self-awareness and Embracing Change: Menopause is a normal part of life because it marks the end of a person's reproductive years and the beginning of a new chapter with opportunities for personal development and self-discovery. Illustrations Took in: The most common way of understanding and overseeing menopausal side effects has shown significant examples taking care of oneself, versatility, and the significance of encouraging groups of people. Challenges Survive Physical and emotional resilience: Many women find that, in spite of the difficulties they face, they emerge stronger and more resilient. Empowerment Through Knowledge: Many women have been able to take control of their health and well-being by learning about menopause and taking proactive measures to manage symptoms. Building People group and

Backing Shared Encounters: Imparting stories and encounters to different ladies going through menopause has made a feeling of local area and common help. Having a support system of friends, family, and medical professionals has been essential for navigating this life change. Key Action items Extensive Comprehension Actual Side effects: Perceiving and dealing with the actual side effects of menopause, from hot glimmers to rest unsettling influences. Emotional well-being: comprehending the effects of menopause on one's emotions and employing methods for preserving one's mental health. Holistic Methods Changes in one's way of life: Supporting one's overall health by eating a well-balanced diet, exercising regularly, and learning ways to manage stress. Alternative Therapies: Investigating complementary and alternative treatments like acupuncture, herbal supplements, and meditation. Prevention-Based Health Care Clinical Therapies: Taking into account clinical medicines like Hormones Replacement Therapy (HRT) and different meds when important. Preventive care emphasizes the significance of routine screenings, examinations, and proactive treatment of persistent conditions. Moving Bits of knowledge Taking Advantage of New Chances Personal Growth: Making the most of this time in one's life to develop oneself, discover new interests, and set new objectives. Career and Retirement: Finding a good balance between work and menopause, thinking about career changes, and making plans for a happy retirement. Positive Perspective Outlook Shift: Review menopause not as an end but rather as a fresh start, loaded up with opportunities for change and self-revelation. Versatility and Strength: Drawing on the internal strength and flexibility created through this excursion to confront future difficulties with certainty. Pushing Ahead with Certainty Aiming for the Future Lifelong learning is the pursuit of knowledge and development through new experiences, hobbies, and education. Wellbeing and Health: Keeping an emphasis on wellbeing and wellbeing through normal activity, a reasonable eating routine, and preventive consideration. Constructing and Keeping up with Emotionally supportive networks Local area Commitment: Remaining associated with help gatherings, companions, and family to share encounters and deal common help. Proficient Direction: Looking for continuous direction from medical services suppliers, specialists, and tutors to successfully explore post-menopausal life. Embracing What's in store Legacy and Impact: Think about the legacy you want to leave behind and the impact you want to have on other people—through mentoring, community service, or personal accomplishments. Living Completely: Embracing every day with appreciation, inspiration, and a promise to make every moment count. Conclusion As you push ahead from "The Menopause Guide," take with you the information, experiences, and devices you have acquired. Embrace this period of existence with certainty, realizing that you have the strength and flexibility to explore any difficulties that come your direction. Keep in mind, menopause isn't an end yet a fresh start, offering open doors for development, self-revelation, and satisfaction. We appreciate you joining us on this journey. May you proceed to flourish and track down delight in this extraordinary phase of life. I look forward to a bright future full of health, happiness, and limitless possibilities.

Chapter 18

Nutrition for Optimal Health

Menopausal symptoms can be managed and overall health can be improved by eating well. This part dives into dietary proposals, key supplements, and down to earth ways to keep a reasonable and nutritious eating routine during menopause. Significance of Nourishment During Menopause Supporting Hormonal Equilibrium Phytoestrogens: These hormone-balancing substances derived from plants can alleviate symptoms like night sweats and hot flashes. Flaxseeds, legumes, and products made from soy are all good sources. Forestalling Weight Gain

Digestion Changes: Hormonal vacillations can dial back digestion, making it simpler to put on weight. A well-balanced diet can help people effectively manage their weight. Bone Wellbeing Calcium and vitamin D are essential for preventing osteoporosis and maintaining bone density. Leafy greens, fortified plant milks, dairy products, and exposure to sunlight are excellent sources. Key Supplements for Menopausal Ladies Calcium Relevance: Crucial to bone health. Sources: Dairy items, invigorated plant milks, mixed greens, almonds, and tofu. D vitamin Significance: Improves calcium assimilation and supports bone wellbeing. Sunlight, fortified foods, fatty fish, and, if necessary, supplements are all sources. Magnesium Significance: Supports muscle capability, energy creation, and bone wellbeing.

Sources: Nuts, seeds, entire grains, and verdant green vegetables. Fatty Acids Omega-3 Significance: Diminishes aggravation, upholds heart wellbeing, and may mitigate state of mind swings. Fat-rich fish like salmon and mackerel, flaxseeds, chia seeds, and walnuts are the sources. Fiber Important: Helps control weight, supports heart health, and aids digestion. Sources: Entire grains, organic products, vegetables, vegetables, and nuts. B Nutrients Significance: Supports energy creation and cerebrum wellbeing. Sources: Entire grains, lean meats, eggs, dairy items, and vegetables. Down to earth Dietary Tips Adjusted Dinners Creation: Go for the gold incorporate an equilibrium of protein, sound fats, and complex carbs. Controlling your portion sizes is an important part of weight management. Hydration

Important: Keeping hydrated can help alleviate symptoms like dry skin and hot flashes. Tips: Stay hydrated throughout the day and avoid alcohol and caffeine. Mindful Diet Procedures: Practice careful eating by focusing on craving and completion signals, eating gradually, and relishing each chomp. Benefits: Forestalls gorging and advances better processing. Solid Eating Options include snacks high in nutrients like yogurt, nuts, fruits, and vegetables. Keep away from: Cutoff handled snacks high in sugar and undesirable fats. A Sample Menu Breakfast Greek yogurt with honey, chia seeds, and fresh berries. Entire grain toast with avocado and a sprinkle of sesame seeds. Lunch Quinoa salad with blended greens, chickpeas, cherry tomatoes, cucumber, and a lemon-tahini dressing. A serving of new natural products. Dinner:

Barbecued salmon with a side of steamed broccoli and yam. A blended green serving of mixed greens with olive oil and balsamic vinegar. Snacks a small amount of almonds. Cut apples with peanut butter. Carrot sticks with hummus. Conclusion An even eating regimen wealthy in fundamental supplements can essentially influence your wellbeing and prosperity during menopause. You can support your overall health and manage symptoms more effectively by making informed dietary choices. Keep in mind, it's never past time to begin focusing on sustenance and receiving the rewards of a sound eating regimen.

Chapter19

Care and Stress Decrease Strategies During menopause, stress management and mental health maintenance are essential. This chapter looks at stress-reduction strategies and mindfulness practices that can help you stay calm, focused, and emotionally balanced. Figuring out Pressure and Menopause Hormonal Impact Hormones and stress: The body's stress response can be affected by hormonal changes during menopause, making stress management more difficult. Influence on Side effects: High feelings of anxiety can intensify menopausal side effects like hot blazes, a sleeping disorder, and emotional episodes. Significance of Stress The board Generally speaking Wellbeing: Constant pressure can prompt different medical problems, including coronary illness, melancholy, and debilitated resistant capability. Personal satisfaction: Viable pressure the board can work on your personal satisfaction, assisting you with feeling more in charge and less wrecked. Practicing Mindfulness What is meditation? The practice of being fully present and engaged in the present moment without judging is known as mindfulness. It has advantages, including the capacity to lessen stress, enhance

mental clarity, and enhance emotional regulation.
Mindfulness-Based Methods Breathing Activities:
Straightforward profound breathing activities can assist with
quieting the brain and lessen pressure. Take a deep breath for
four, hold it for four, and then exhale for four. Body Sweep:
This training includes intellectually examining your body from
head to toe, taking note of areas of pressure and intentionally
loosening them up. Careful Contemplation: Put away
opportunity every day for careful reflection. Center around
your breath, a mantra, or a serene picture to focus your brain.
Including Mindfulness in Everyday Life Mindful eating means
taking in every bite and paying attention to how it tastes, feels,
and smells. Careful Strolling: Go for a stroll in nature,
focusing on the sights, sounds, and sensations around you. Day
to day Everyday practice: Coordinate care into day to day
undertakings, like washing dishes, by zeroing in completely on
the action within reach. Stress Decrease Methods Exercise
Benefits: Engaging in physical activity has been shown to
improve mood and lower levels of stress hormones and
endorphins. Types: Integrate vigorous activities, strength
preparing, yoga, or jujitsu into your daily schedule. Unwinding
Strategies Moderate Muscle Unwinding: This method includes
straining and afterward leisurely loosening up each muscle

bunch in the body. Directed Symbolism: Imagine a tranquil scene or experience to assist with decreasing pressure and advance unwinding. Journaling: Expounding on your viewpoints and sentiments can be a restorative method for handling feelings and diminish pressure. Social Help Interface with Others: Construct areas of strength for an organization of companions, family, and partners. Seek Professional Assistance: If stress becomes overwhelming, you might want to talk to a therapist or counselor for more help. Leisure activities and Interests Participate in Exercises: Seek after leisure activities and exercises that give pleasure and unwinding, like perusing, cultivating, or making. Inventive Outlets: Put yourself out there through imaginative outlets like work of art, composing, or music. Conclusion During menopause, incorporating mindfulness and techniques for reducing stress into your daily routine can significantly enhance your mental and emotional well-being. By remaining present, overseeing pressure successfully, and sustaining your close to home wellbeing, you can explore this progress effortlessly and certainty. Keep in mind that taking care of your mind and body go hand in hand. Embrace these practices to upgrade your general personal satisfaction.

Conclusion

As "The Menopause Guide" comes to an end, it's important to think back on the amazing journey you've taken. Menopause is a characteristic, groundbreaking stage in a lady's life, loaded up with the two difficulties and open doors. This guide has planned to give you complete information, viable counsel, and everyday reassurance to explore this progress with certainty and effortlessness. Accepting Change Menopause denotes the finish of one section and the start of another, offering a special chance for development and self-disclosure. The way you feel about this phase can change if you accept these changes with a positive attitude. By getting it and dealing with the physical and profound side effects, you can assume command over your wellbeing and prosperity. Strengthening Through Information Power is knowledge. By teaching yourself about the different parts of menopause — from hormonal changes to close to home prosperity, from clinical medicines to elective treatments — you are better prepared to settle on informed choices that suit your singular requirements. You can approach menopause with confidence and preparedness thanks to this empowerment. Building Solid Emotionally supportive networks One of the main focus points from this guide is the significance of building and keeping up areas of strength for frameworks. Whether through family, companions, medical services suppliers, or care groups, having an organization of individuals who comprehend and uphold you can improve things significantly. Sharing your encounters and gaining from others makes a feeling of local area and common strengthening. Embracing an All encompassing Methodology A comprehensive way to deal with overseeing menopause — one that incorporates adjusted sustenance, standard actual work, stress the executives, and elective treatments — can essentially improve your personal satisfaction. You can make this transition go more smoothly and keep your overall health by focusing on your physical and emotional well-being at the same time. Looking Ahead The excursion through menopause isn't just about overseeing side effects; it's additionally about anticipating new open doors and embracing the future with good faith. This period of life offers the opportunity to rediscover yourself, put forth new objectives, and investigate new interests. The options are endless, and they can include pursuing new hobbies, changing careers, or furthering one's education. Persistent Development and Learning Menopause is a time of continuous learning and development. Keep your mind open to new opportunities and keep your curiosity alive.

This mentality will assist you with adjusting to changes and track down happiness and satisfaction in this phase of life. Recognizing Your Resilience and Strength At long last, pause for a minute to commend your solidarity and strength. Your journey is a testament to your bravery and perseverance as you navigate menopause. You have the instruments, information, and support to flourish, and this guide has planned to be a sidekick en route. A Future Packed with Opportunities As you push ahead, recall that menopause is only one piece of your life's process. Embrace it as a period of restoration and change. You have the strength and insight to make the most of the many opportunities that lie ahead. Much obliged to you for permitting "The Menopause Guide" to be essential for your excursion. May you keep on flourishing, develop, and track down satisfaction in each step of this extraordinary phase of life. Here's to a future loaded up with wellbeing, bliss, and vast conceivable outcomes.